Plant-Based Diet for Beginners

A Complete Collection of Amazing Meals Recipes to Start Your Diet and Improve Your Skills

Carl Brady

Table of Contents

Spicy Cajun Boiled Peanuts

Servings: 15 Preparation time: 8 hours and 5 minutes

Ingredients:

5 pounds of peanuts, raw and in shells

6-ounce of dry crab boil

4-ounce of jalapeno peppers, sliced

2-ounce of vegetable broth

Directions:

Take a 6-quarts slow cooker place the ingredients in it and cover it with water. Stir properly and cover the top. Plug in the slow cooker; adjust the cooking time to 8 hours and let it cook on the low heat setting or until the peanuts are soft and floats on top of the cooking liquid. Drain the nuts and serve right away.

Yogurt Soup with Rice

Preparation Time: 15 minutes Cooking Time: 48 minutes

Servings: 6

Ingredients:

½ cup brown rice, rinsed and drained

1 egg

4 cups yogurt

3 tbsp. rice flour

3 cups water

½ cup mint, chopped

½ cup cilantro, chopped

½ cup dill, chopped

½ cup parsley, chopped

2 cups arugula

Salt to taste

Directions:

Combine the rice, egg, yogurt and flour in a pot. Put it over medium heat and cook for 1 minute, stirring frequently. Pour in the water and increase heat to boil. Reduce heat and simmer for 45 minutes. Add the arugula, herbs and salt. Cook for 2 minutes. Add more water to adjust consistency.

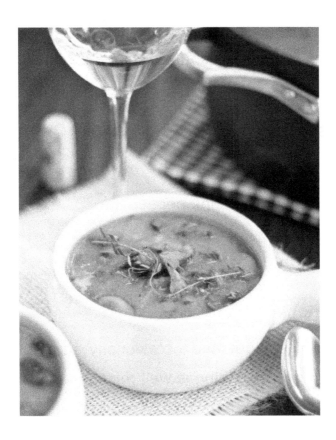

Green cheese sauce and nacho chile

Preparation Time: 30minutes

Ingredients:

1 cup raw cashews, soaked in 2 cups of water for 2-4 hours, drain and rinse

1/4 cup roasted red pepper, diced (glass is fine)

1/4 cup green chilies, diced (cans are fine)

2 tablespoons yeast flakes

2 teaspoons lemon juice

1 cup of water

1/4 teaspoon cayenne pepper

1/2 teaspoon sea salt

Directions:

Mix until smooth and occasionally scrape the sides to make sure everything is well mixed.

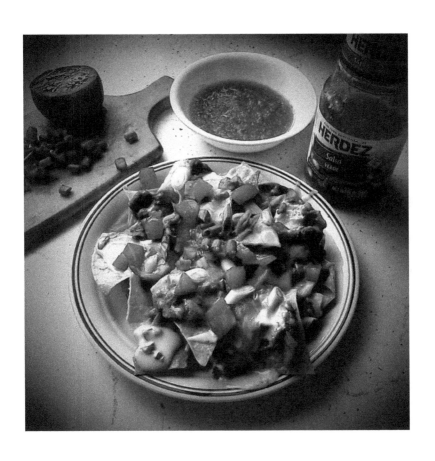

Spicy Black Bean Burgers

Total Preparation & Cooking time: 25 min. Servings: 6

Ingredients:

1 minced jalapeno pepper, small

1/2 cup flour

2 minced garlic cloves

1/2 tsp. oregano, dried

1 diced onion, small

1/2 cup corn niblets

2 cups mashed black beans, canned

1/4 cup breadcrumbs

2 tsp. minced parsley (optional)

1/4 tsp. cumin

1 tbsp. olive oil

1/2 diced red pepper, medium

 2 tsp. chili powder

1/2 tsp. salt

Directions:

To coat, set aside the flour on a small plate. Sauté the garlic, onion, hot peppers, and oregano in oil on medium-high heat settings in a medium saucepan, until the onions are translucent. Put in the peppers & sauté until pepper is tender, approximately 2 more minutes. Keep it aside. Use a fork or potato masher to mash the black beans in a large bowl. Stir in the vegetables cumin, breadcrumbs, chili powder, parsley and salt. Mix well and divide to make 6 patties. Coat each side of the patty by laying it down in the flour. Cook the patties on a lightly oiled frying pan until browned on either sides or approximately 10 minutes on medium-high heat.

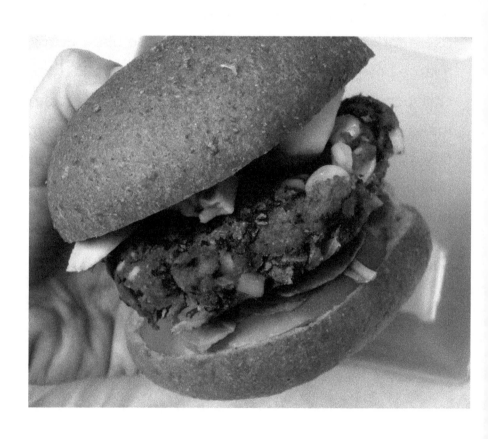

Vodka Cream Sauce

Preparation time: 5 minutes Cooking time: 5 minutes
Servings: 1

Ingredients:

1/4 cup cashews, unsalted , soaked in warm water for 15 minutes

24-ounce marinara sauce

2 tablespoons vodka

1/4 cup water

Directions:

Drain the cashews, transfer them in a food processor, pour in water, and blend for 2 minutes until smooth. Tip the mixture in a pot, stir in pasta sauce and vodka and simmer for 3 minutes over medium heat until done, stirring constantly. Serve sauce over pasta.

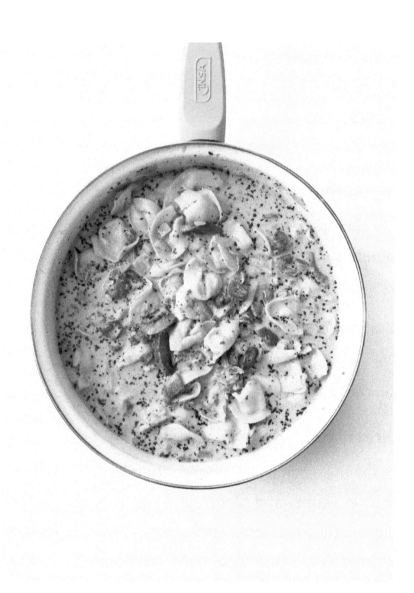

Hot Sauce

Preparation time: 5 minutes Cooking time: 0 minute

Servings: 16

Ingredients:

4 cloves of garlic, peeled

15 Hot peppers, de-stemmed, chopped

1/2 teaspoon. coriander

1/2 teaspoon. sea salt

1/2 teaspoon. red chili powder

1/2 of lime, zested

1/4 teaspoon. cumin

1/2 lime, juiced

1 cup apple cider vinegar

Directions:

Place all the ingredients in the order in a food processor or blender and then pulse for 3 to 5 minutes at high speed until smooth. Tip the sauce in a bowl and then serve.

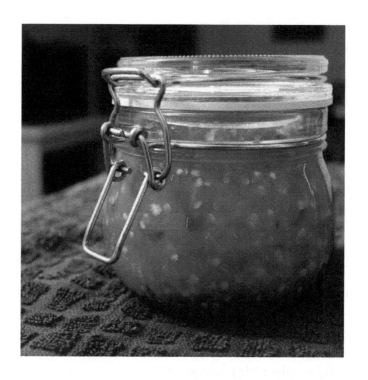

Barbecue Sauce

Preparation time: 5 minutes Cooking time: 0 minute Servings: 16

Ingredients:

8 ounces tomato sauce

1 teaspoon garlic powder

¼ teaspoon ground black pepper

1/2 teaspoon. sea salt

2 Tablespoons Dijon mustard

3 packets stevia

1 teaspoon molasses

1 Tablespoon apple cider vinegar

2 Tablespoons tamari

1 teaspoon liquid aminos

Directions:

Take a medium bowl, place all the ingredients in it, and stir until combined. Serve straight away

Bolognese Sauce

Preparation time: 10 minutes Cooking time: 45 minutes

Servings: 8

Ingredients:

½ of small green bell pepper, chopped

1 stalk of celery, chopped

1 small carrot, chopped

1 medium white onion, peeled, chopped

2 teaspoons minced garlic

1/2 teaspoon crushed red pepper flakes

3 tablespoons olive oil

8-ounce tempeh, crumbled

8 ounces white mushrooms, chopped

1/2 cup dried red lentils

28-ounce crushed tomatoes

28-ounce whole tomatoes, chopped

1 teaspoon dried oregano

1/2 teaspoon fennel seed

1/2 teaspoon ground black pepper

1/2 teaspoon salt

1 teaspoon dried basil

1/4 cup chopped parsley

1 bay leaf

6-ounce tomato paste

1 cup dry red wine

Directions:

Take a Dutch oven, place it over medium heat, add oil, and when hot, add the first six ingredients, stir and cook for 5 minutes until sauté. Then switch heat to medium-high level, add two ingredients after olive oil, stir and cook for 3 minutes. Switch heat to medium-low level, stir in tomato paste, and continue cooking for 2 minutes. Add remaining ingredients except for lentils, stir and bring the mixture to boil. Switch heat to the low level, simmer sauce for 10 minutes, covering the pan partially, then add lentils and continue cooking for 20 minutes until tender. Serve sauce with cooked pasta.

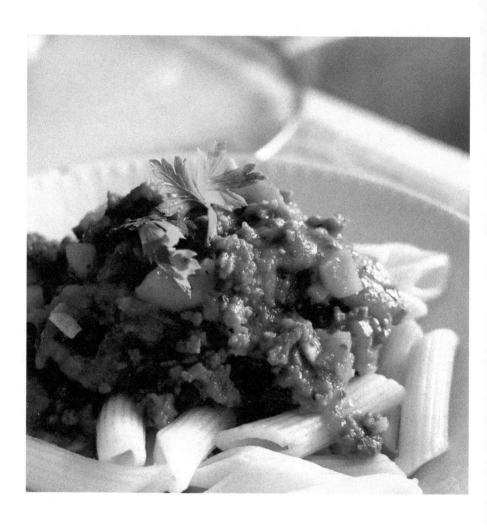

Alfredo Sauce

Preparation time: 5 minutes Cooking time: 0 minute
Servings: 4

Ingredients:

1 cup cashews, unsalted, soaked in warm water for 15 minutes

1 teaspoon minced garlic

1/4 teaspoon ground black pepper

1/3 teaspoon salt

1/4 cup nutritional yeast

2 tablespoons tamari

2 tablespoons olive oil

4 tablespoons water

Directions:

Drain the cashews, transfer them into a food processor, add remaining ingredients in it, and pulse for 3 minutes until thick sauce comes together. Serve straight away.

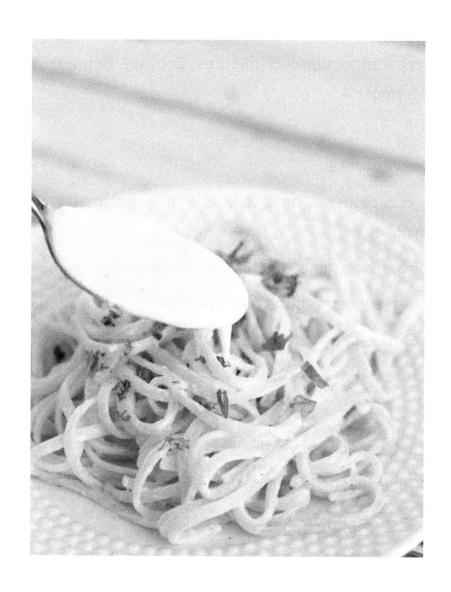

Garden Pesto

Preparation time: 5 minutes Cooking time: 0 minute

Servings: 10

Ingredients:

1/4 cup pistachios, shelled

3/4 cup parsley leaves

1 cup cilantro leaves

½ teaspoon minced garlic

1/4 cup mint leaves

1 cup basil leaves

¼ teaspoon ground black pepper

1/3 teaspoon salt

1/2 cup olive oil

1 1/2 teaspoons miso

2 teaspoons lemon juice

Directions: Place all the ingredients in the order in a food processor or blender and then pulse for 3 to 5 minutes at high speed until smooth. Tip the pesto in a bowl and then serve.

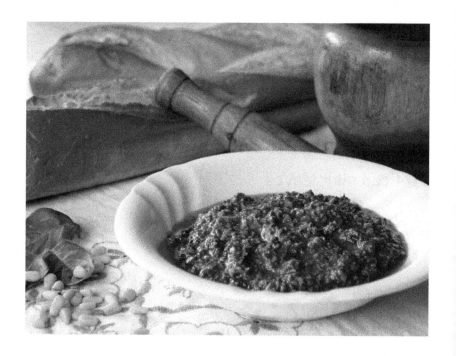

Cilantro and Parsley Hot Sauce

Preparation time: 5 minutes Cooking time: 0 minute

Servings: 4

Ingredients:

2 cups of parsley and cilantro leaves with stems

4 Thai bird chilies, destemmed, deseeded, torn

2 teaspoons minced garlic

1 teaspoon salt

1/4 teaspoon coriander seed, ground

1/4 teaspoon ground black pepper

1/2 teaspoon cumin seeds, ground

3 green cardamom pods, toasted, ground

1/2 cup olive oil

Directions:

Take a spice blender or a food processor, place all the ingredients in it, and process for 5 minutes until the smooth paste comes together. Serve straight away.

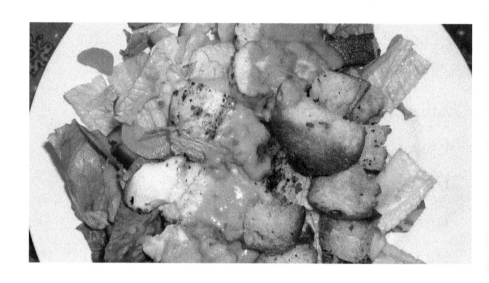

Sushi Bowl

Serves: 1 Time: 40 Minutes

Ingredients:

½ Cup Edamame Beans, Shelled & Fresh

¾ Cup Brown Rice, Cooked

½ Cup Spinach, Chopped

¼ Cup Bell Pepper, Sliced

¼ Cup Avocado, Sliced

¼ Cup Cilantro, Fresh & Chopped

1 Scallion, Chopped

¼ Nori Sheet

1-2 Tablespoons Tamari

1 Tablespoon Sesame Seeds, Optional

Directions:

Steam your edamame beans, and then assemble your edamame, rice, avocado, spinach, cilantro, scallions and bell pepper into a bowl. Cut the nori into ribbons, sprinkling it on top, drizzling with tamari and sesame seeds before serving. Interesting Facts: Avocados are known as miracle fruits in the world of Veganism. They are true super-fruit and incredibly beneficial. They are one of the best things to eat if you are looking to incorporate more fatty acids in your diet. They are also loaded with 20 various minerals and vitamins. Plus, they are easy to incorporate into dishes all throughout the day!

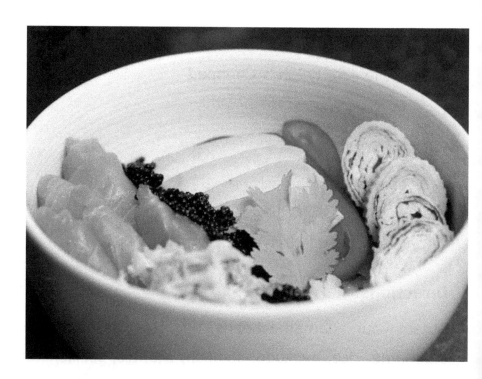

Corn and Potato Chowder

Preparation time: 5 minutes Cooking time: 35 minutes

Servings: 4

Ingredients:

2 ears of corn

10 ounces tofu, extra-firm, drained cubed

1 1/2 cups frozen corn kernels

1/4 medium onion, peeled, chopped

3 medium potatoes, peeled, cubed

1/4 medium red bell pepper, cored, chopped

¼ cup cilantro, chopped

2/3 teaspoon salt

1/4 cup coconut cream

7 cups of vegetable broth

Directions:

Prepare the ears of corn and for this, remove their skin and husk, then cut each corn into four pieces and place them in a large pot. Place the pot over medium-high heat, add cilantro, onion and bell pepper, pour in the broth, bring the mixture to boil, then switch heat to medium level and cook for 20 minutes until corn pieces are tender. Add potatoes, cook for 8 minutes until fork tender, then add tofu and kernels, simmer for 5 minutes and taste to adjust seasoning. Remove pot from heat, stir in cream until combined and serve straight away.

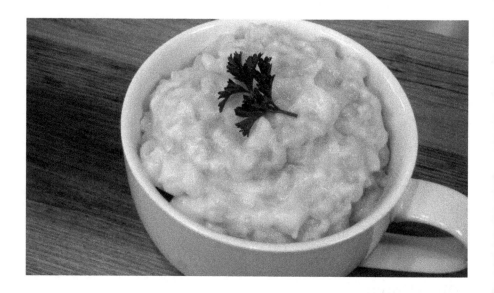

Red Pepper and Tomato Soup

Preparation time: 10 minutes Cooking time: 40 minutes
Servings: 4

Ingredients:

2 carrots, peeled, chopped

1 1/4 pounds red bell peppers, deseeded, sliced into quarters

1/2 of medium red onion, peeled, sliced into thin wedges

16 ounces small tomatoes, halved

1 tablespoon chopped basil

1/2 teaspoon salt

2 cups vegetable broth

Directions:

Switch on the oven, then set it to 450 degrees F and let it preheat. Then place all the vegetables in a single on a baking sheet lined with foil and roast for 40 minutes until the skins of peppers are slightly charred. When done, remove the baking sheet from the oven, let them cool for

10 minutes, then peel the peppers and transfer all the vegetables into a blender. Add basil and salt to the vegetables, pour in the broth, and puree the vegetables until smooth. Serve straight away.

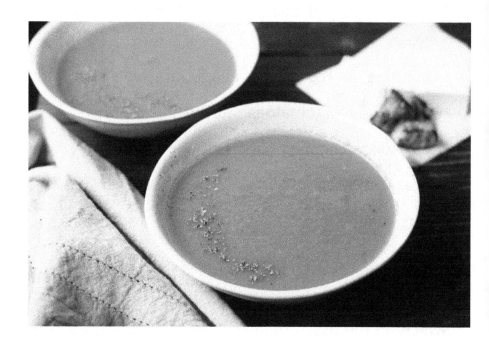

Wonton Soup

Preparation time: 15 minutes Cooking time: 10 minutes

Servings: 4

Ingredients:

For the Soup: 4 cups vegetable broth

2 green onions, chopped

For the Wontons Filling: 1 cup chopped mushrooms

1/4 cup walnuts, chopped

1 green onion, chopped

1/2 inch of ginger, grated

½ teaspoon minced garlic

1 tablespoon rice vinegar

2 teaspoons soy sauce

1 teaspoon brown sugar

20 Vegan Wonton Wrappers

Directions:

Prepare wonton filling and for this, take a bowl, place all the ingredients in it, except for wrapper and toss until well combined. Place a wonton wrapper on working space, place 1 teaspoon of prepared filling in the middle, then brush some water at the edges, fold over to shape like a half-moon, and seal the wrappers by pinching the edges. Take a large pot, place it over medium-high heat, add broth, and bring it to boil. Then drop prepared wontons in it, one at a time, and boil for 5 minutes. When cooked, garnish the soup with green onions and serve.

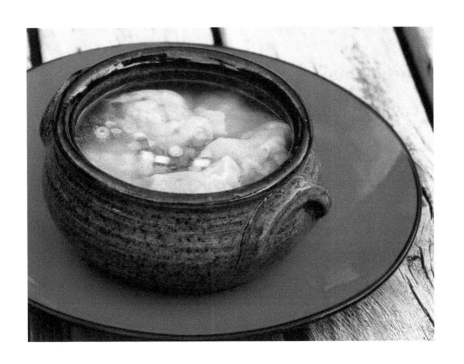

Broccoli Cheese Soup

Preparation time: 10 minutes Cooking time: 15 minutes

Servings: 4

Ingredients:

1 medium potato, peeled, diced

2 ribs celery, diced

1 medium white onion, peeled, diced

2 medium yellow summer squash, diced

1 medium carrot, peeled, diced

6 cups chopped broccoli florets

1 teaspoon minced garlic

1 bay leaf

1/3 teaspoon ground black pepper

¼ cup nutritional yeast

1 tablespoon lemon juice

2 tablespoons apple cider vinegar

½ cup cashews

3 cups of water

Directions:

Take a large pot, place it over medium-high heat, add all the vegetables in it, except for florets, add bay leaf, pour in water and bring the mixture to boil. Then switch heat to medium-low and simmer for 10 minutes until vegetables are tender. Meanwhile, place broccoli florets in another pot, place it over medium-low heat and cook for 4 minutes or more until broccoli has steamed. When done, remove broccoli from the pot, reserve 1 cup of its liquid, and set aside until required. When vegetables have cooked, remove the bay leaf, add remaining ingredients in it, reserving broccoli and its liquid, and then puree the soup by using an immersion blender until smooth. Then add steamed broccoli along with its liquid, stir well and serve straight away.

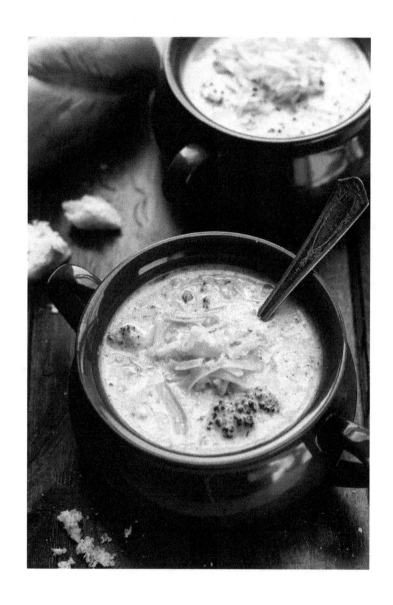

Vegan Pho

Preparation time: 5 minutes Cooking time: 15 minutes Servings: 6

Ingredients:

1 package of wide rice noodles, cooked

1 medium white onion, peeled, quartered

2 teaspoons minced garlic

1 inch of ginger, sliced into coins

8 cups vegetable broth

3 whole cloves

2 tablespoons soy sauce

3 whole star anise

1 cinnamon stick

3 cups of water

For Toppings:

Basil as needed for topping

Chopped green onions as needed for topping

Ming beans as needed for topping

Hot sauce as needed for topping

Lime wedges for serving

Directions:

Take a large pot, place it over medium-high heat, add all the ingredients for soup in it, except for soy sauce and broth, and bring it to boil. Then switch heat to medium-low level, simmer the soup for 30 minutes and then stir in soy sauce. When done, distribute cooked noodles into bowls, top with soup, then top with toppings and serve.

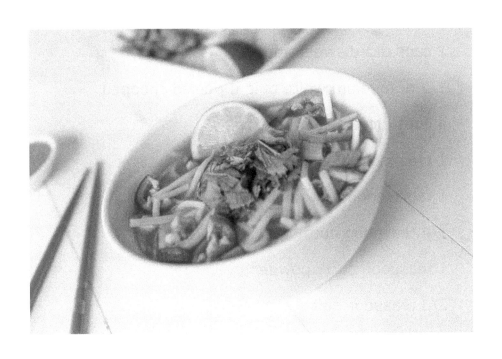

Curried Apple and Sweet Potato Soup

Preparation time: 10 minutes Cooking time: 38 minutes
Servings: 6

Ingredients:

2 cups diced sweet apples

1/2 of medium white onion, peeled chopped

4 cups diced sweet potatoes

1 teaspoon minced garlic

1 tablespoon grated ginger

1/4 teaspoon nutmeg

1 teaspoon curry powder

2/3 teaspoon salt

1/3 teaspoon ground black pepper

1/2 teaspoon cinnamon

1 tablespoon olive oil

2 cups apple cider

1 cup vegetable stock

1 cup coconut milk, unsweetened

For Garnish: 1/2 cup baked apple chips 1/4 cup toasted pumpkin seeds 1/4 cup coconut milk, unsweetened

Directions:

Take a large pot, place it over medium-high heat and when hot, add oil and onion and cook 5 minutes until translucent. Add garlic and ginger, stir in all the spices, then add sweet potatoes and cook for 4 minutes until sauté. Switch heat to medium-low level, add apples, pour in milk, stock, and cider coconut and simmer 25 minutes until vegetables are softened. Puree the soup by using an immersion blender, season with salt and black pepper, and distribute into bowls. Top with garnishing and then serve.

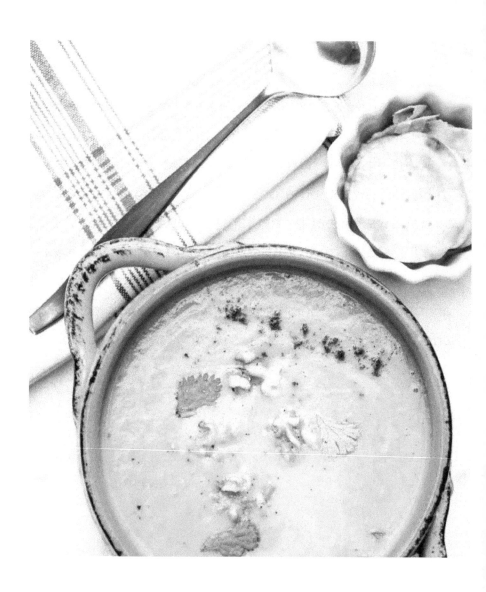

Lasagna Soup

Preparation time: 5 minutes Cooking time: 5 hours and 12 minutes Servings: 6

Ingredients:

For the Lasagna Soup:

3/4 cup dried brown lentils

1 medium white onion, peeled, diced

3 cups chopped spinach leaves

14 ounces crushed tomatoes

14 ounces diced tomatoes

1 ½ teaspoon minced garlic

1 teaspoon dried basil

1 teaspoon dried oregano

8 lasagna noodles, broken into pieces

4 1/2 cups vegetable broth

For the Vegan Pesto Ricotta:

1/4 pound tofu, extra firm, drained

1 cup cashews, soaked, drained

2/3 teaspoon salt

1/3 teaspoon ground black pepper

4 tablespoons pesto, vegan

1 tablespoon lemon juice

1/4 cup almond milk

Directions:

Prepare the lasagna soup and for this, switch on the slow cooker, add lentils, onion, and garlic in it, stir in basil and oregano, pour in broth, and stir until mixed. Shut the slow cooker with lid and cook for 2 hours at a high heat setting. Meanwhile, prepare the pesto ricotta, and for this, place cashews in a blender, add milk and pulse until smooth. Then tofu, pulse until mixture resembles ricotta cheese, then tip it in a bowl and stir in remaining ingredients until combined, set aside until required. Then stir in all the tomatoes, continue cooking for 3 hours at high heat setting, add noodles and spinach, stir until mixed and cook for 12 minutes until spinach leaves have wilted. When done, season the soup with salt and black pepper and then serve with prepared pesto ricotta.

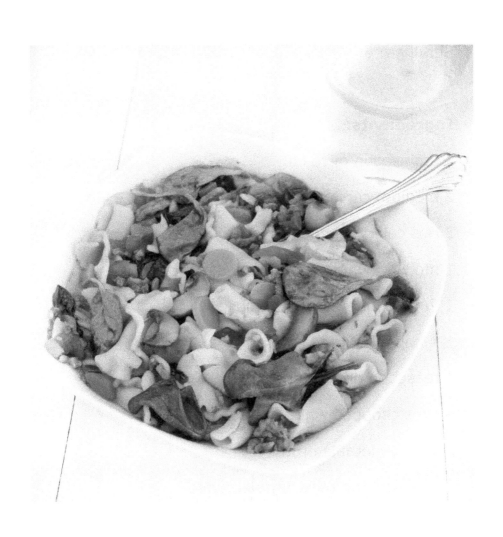

Potato and Corn Chowder

Preparation time: 5 minutes Cooking time: 16 minutes
Servings: 6

Ingredients:

1 tablespoon olive oil

2 medium carrots, peeled, chopped

2 ribs celery, chopped

1 medium white onion, peeled, chopped

1 ½ teaspoon minced garlic

1/4 cup all-purpose flour

1 teaspoon dried thyme

4 cups chopped white potatoes

2 cups vegetable broth

2 cups almond milk, unsweetened

3 tablespoons nutritional yeast

1 cup frozen corn kernels

1 teaspoon salt

1/4 teaspoon ground black pepper

Directions:

Take a large pot, place it over medium-high heat, add oil and when hot, add onion, carrots, celery, and garlic and cook for 5 minutes until golden brown. Then sprinkle with flour and thyme, stir until coated, cook for 1 minute until the flour has browned, then add yeast, potatoes, milk, and broth and stir until mixed. Bring the mixture to simmer, cook for 8 minutes until tender, then add corn and season the soup with salt and black pepper. Serve straight away.

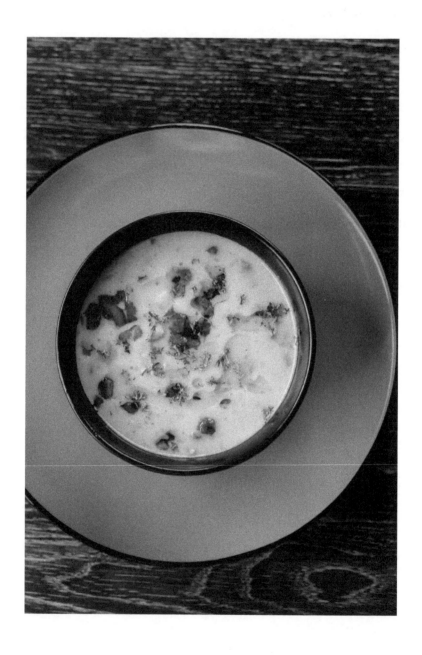

Spanish Chickpea and Sweet Potato Stew

Preparation time: 5 minutes Cooking time: 35 minutes

Servings: 4

Ingredients:

14 ounces cooked chickpeas

1 small sweet potato, peeled, cut into

½-inch cubes

1 medium red onion, sliced

3 ounces baby spinach

14 ounces crushed tomatoes

2 teaspoons minced garlic

1 teaspoon salt

1 1/2 teaspoons ground cumin

2 teaspoons harissa paste

2 teaspoons maple syrup

½ teaspoon ground black pepper

2 teaspoons sugar

1 tablespoon olive oil

1/2 cup vegetable stock

2 tablespoons chopped parsley

1 ounce slivered almonds, toasted

Brown rice, cooked, for serving

Directions:

Take a large saucepan, place it over low heat, add oil and when hot, add onion and garlic and cook for 5 minutes. Then add sweet potatoes, season with cumin, stir in harissa paste and cook for 2 minutes until toasted. Switch heat to medium-low level, add tomatoes and chickpeas, pour in vegetable stock, stir in maple syrup and sugar and simmer for 25 minutes until potatoes have softened, stirring every 10 minutes. Then add spinach, cook for 1 minute until its leaves have wilted, and season with salt and black pepper. When done, distribute cooked rice between bowls, top with stew, garnish with parsley and almonds and serve.

Sweet Potato, Kale and Peanut Stew

Preparation time: 10 minutes Cooking time: 45 minutes

Servings: 3

Ingredients:

1/4 cup red lentils

2 medium sweet potatoes, peeled, cubed

1 medium white onion, peeled, diced

1 cup kale, chopped

2 tomatoes, diced

1/4 cup chopped green onion

1 teaspoon minced garlic

1 inch of ginger, grated

2 tablespoons toasted peanuts

¼ teaspoon ground black pepper

1 teaspoon ground cumin

1/2 teaspoon turmeric

1/8 teaspoon cayenne pepper

1 tablespoon peanut butter

1 1/2 cups vegetable broth

2 teaspoons coconut oil

Directions:

Take a medium pot, place it medium heat, add oil and when it melts, add onions and cook for 5 minutes. Then stir in ginger and garlic, cook for 2 minutes until fragrant, add lentils and potatoes along with all the spices, and stir until mixed. Stir in tomatoes, pour in the broth, bring the mixture to boil, then switch heat to the low level and simmer for 30 minutes until cooked. Then stir in peanut butter until incorporated and then puree by using an immersion blender until half-pureed. Return stew over low heat, stir in kale, cook for 5 minutes until its leaves wilts, and then season with black pepper and salt. Garnish the stew with peanuts and green onions and then serve.

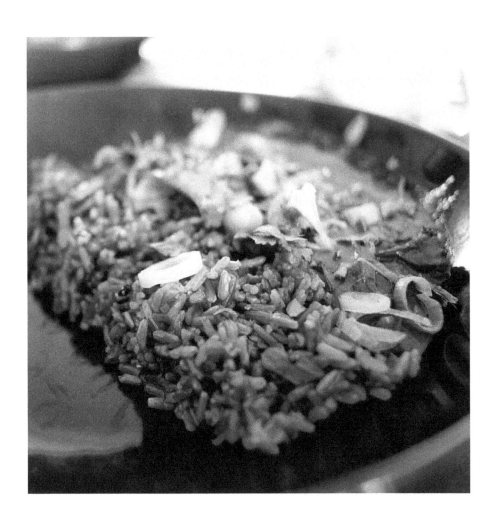

White Bean and Cabbage Stew

Preparation time: 5 minutes Cooking time: 8 hours Servings: 4

Ingredients:

3 cups cooked great northern beans

1.5 pounds potatoes, peeled, cut in large dice

1 large white onion, peeled, chopped

½ head of cabbage, chopped

3 ribs celery, chopped

4 medium carrots, peeled, sliced

14.5 ounces diced tomatoes

1/3 cup pearled barley

1 teaspoon minced garlic

½ teaspoon ground black pepper

1 bay leaf

1 teaspoon dried thyme

½ teaspoon crushed rosemary

1 teaspoon salt

½ teaspoon caraway seeds

1 tablespoon chopped parsley

8 cups vegetable broth

Directions:

Switch on the slow cooker, then add all the ingredients except for salt, parsley, tomatoes, and beans and stir until mixed. Shut the slow cooker with lid, and cook for 7 hours at low heat setting until cooked. Then stir in remaining ingredients, stir until combined and continue cooking for 1 hour. Serve straight away

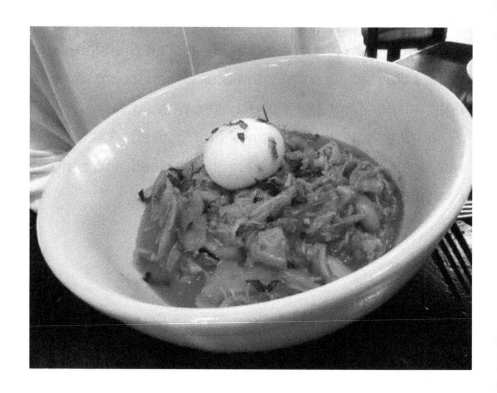

Fennel and Chickpeas Provençal

Preparation time: 10 minutes Cooking time: 50 minutes

Servings: 4

Ingredients:

15 ounces cooked chickpeas 3

 fennel bulbs, sliced

1 medium onion, peeled, sliced

15 ounces diced tomatoes

10 black olives, pitted, cured

10 Kalamata olives, pitted

1 ½ teaspoon minced garlic

1 teaspoon salt

1/8 teaspoon ground black pepper

1 teaspoon Herbes de Provence

1/2 teaspoon red pepper flakes

2 tablespoons olive oil

1/2 cup water

2 tablespoons chopped parsley

Directions:

Take a saucepan, place it over medium-high heat, add oil and when hot, add onion, fennel, and garlic and cook for 20 minutes until softened. Then add remaining ingredients except for olives and chickpeas, bring the mixture to boil, switch heat to medium-low level and simmer for 15 minutes. Then add remaining ingredients, cook for 10 minutes until hot, garnish stew with parsley and serve.

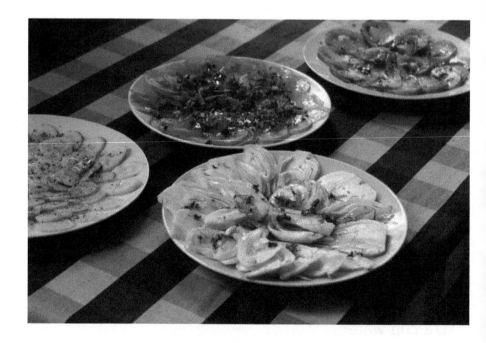

Kimchi Stew

Preparation time: 10 minutes Cooking time: 25 minutes

Servings: 4

Ingredients:

1 pound tofu, extra-firm, pressed, cut into

1-inch pieces

4 cups napa cabbage kimchi, vegan, chopped

1 small white onion, peeled, diced

2 cups sliced shiitake mushroom caps

1 ½ teaspoon minced garlic

2 tablespoons soy sauce

2 tablespoons olive oil, divided

4 cups vegetable broth

2 tablespoons chopped scallions

Directions:

Take a large pot, place it over medium heat, add 1 tablespoon oil and when hot, add tofu pieces in a single layer and cook for 10 minutes until browned on all sides. When cooked, transfer tofu pieces to a plate, add remaining oil to the pot and when hot, add onion and cook for 5 minutes until soft. Stir in garlic, cook for 1 minute until fragrant, stir in kimchi, continue cooking for 2 minutes, then add mushrooms and pour in broth. Switch heat to medium-high level, bring the mixture to boil, then switch heat to medium-low level and simmer for 10 minutes until mushrooms are softened. Stir in tofu, taste to adjust seasoning, and garnish with scallions. Serve straight away.

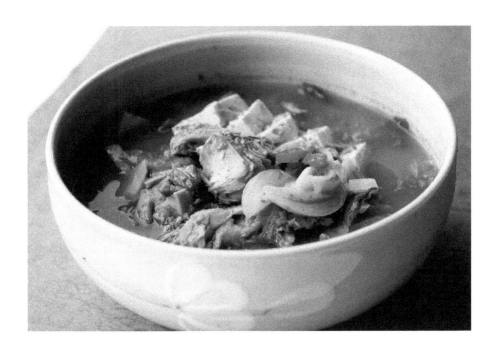

Oatmeal Pancake

Preparation Time: 10 minutes Cooking Time: 30 minutes

Servings: 8

Ingredients:

½ cup blueberries

3 bananas, sliced

2 tsp. lemon juice

¼ cup maple syrup

¼ tsp. ground cinnamon

1 cup flour

2 tsp. baking powder

½ tsp. baking soda

½ cup rolled oats

Salt to taste

1 egg, beaten

1 cup buttermilk

1 tsp. vanilla

1 tbsp. olive oil

Directions:

Toss the blueberries and bananas in lemon juice, maple syrup and cinnamon. Set aside. In a bowl, mix the flour, baking powder, baking soda, oats and salt. In another bowl, combine the egg, milk and vanilla. Slowly add the second bowl mixture into the first one. Mix well. Pour the oil into a pan over medium heat. Pour 4 tablespoons of the batter and cook for 2 minutes per side. Repeat with the remaining batter. Serve the pancakes with the fruits.

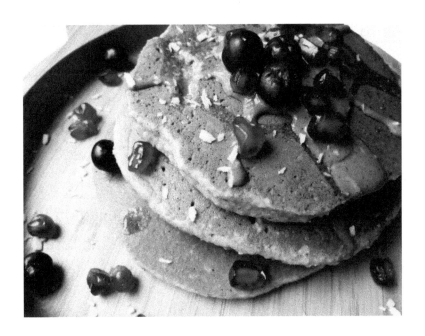

Avocado & Egg Salad on Toasted Bread

Preparation Time: 5 minutes Cooking Time: 0 minute

Servings: 2

Ingredients:

½ avocado

1 tsp. lemon juice

2 hard-boiled egg, chopped

2 tbsp. celery, chopped

Salt to taste

1 tsp. hot sauce

2 slices whole-wheat bread, toasted

Directions:

Mash the avocado in a bowl. Stir in the lemon juice, egg, celery, salt and hot sauce. Spread the mixture on top of the toasted bread.

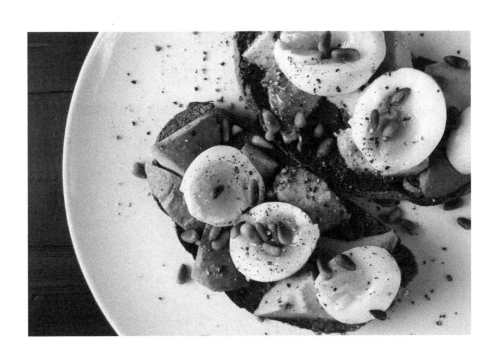

Cauliflower and Horseradish Soup

Preparation time: 5 minutes Cooking time: 20 minutes
Servings: 4

Ingredients:

2 medium potatoes, peeled, chopped

1 medium cauliflower, florets and stalk chopped

1 medium white onion, peeled, chopped

1 teaspoon minced garlic

2/3 teaspoon salt

1/3 teaspoon ground black pepper

4 teaspoons horseradish sauce

1 teaspoon dried thyme

3 cups vegetable broth

1 cup coconut milk, unsweetened

Directions: Place all the vegetables in a large pan, place it over medium-high heat, add thyme, pour in broth and milk and bring the mixture to boil. Then switch heat to medium level, simmer the soup for 15 minutes and remove the pan from heat. Puree the soup by using an immersion blender until smooth, season with salt and black pepper, and serve straight away.

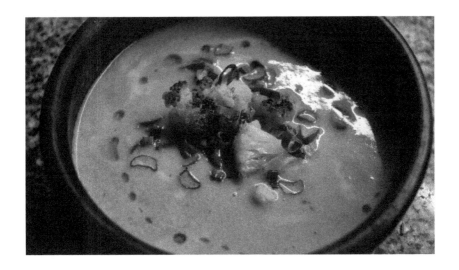

Chickpea Noodle Soup

Preparation time: 5 minutes Cooking time: 18 minutes Servings: 6

Ingredients:

1 cup cooked chickpeas

8 ounces rotini noodles, whole-wheat

4 celery stalks, sliced

2 medium white onions, peeled, chopped

4 medium carrots, peeled, sliced

2 teaspoons minced garlic

8 sprigs of thyme

1 teaspoon salt

1/3 teaspoon ground black pepper

1 bay leaf

2 tablespoons olive oil

2 quarts of vegetable broth

¼ cup chopped fresh parsley

Directions: Take a large pot, place it over medium heat, add oil and when hot, add all the vegetables, stir in garlic, thyme and bay leaf and cook for 5 minutes until vegetables are golden and sauté. Then pour in broth stir and bring the mixture to boil. Add chickpeas and noodles into boiling soup, continue cooking for 8 minutes until noodles are tender, and then season soup with salt and black pepper. Garnish with parsley and serve straight away.

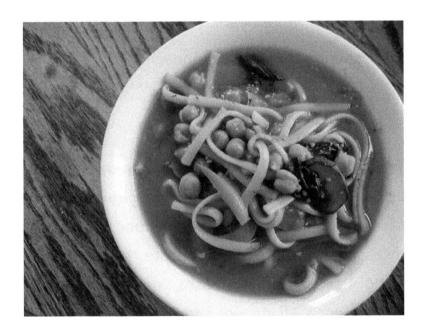

Quinoa Pepper Burgers

Preparation time: 10 minutes Cooking time: 30 minutes

Servings 6–8 burgers

Ingredients:

2/3 cup uncooked quinoa

3 cups water or vegetable broth

4 roasted red bell peppers

1 cup canned white beans

2 tablespoons chopped coriander

Salt, pepper (to taste)

Directions: Bring 3 cups water/broth to a boil. Add quinoa, remove from heat and allow quinoa to absorb all of the liquid. Combine the bell pepper and beans in food processor and pulse until a paste forms. In a medium mixing bowl, combine paste, quinoa, coriander, and salt/pepper. 3. Using wet hands, form the mixture into a burger shape. Add one tablespoon of olive oil to frying pan and heat over medium. Cook burgers on each side 7 minutes, until crispy.

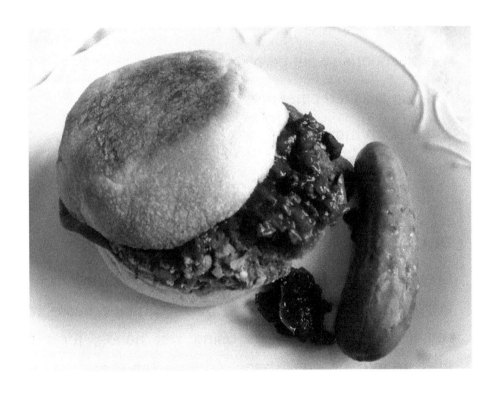

Tropical Island Burgers

Preparation time: 10 minutes Cooking time: 30 minutes

Servings 6–8 burgers

Ingredients:

3 cups canned black beans, rinsed and drained

1/2 cup rolled oats

4 tablespoons sweet corn

1/4 cup crushed pineapple

1 teaspoon mustard

Salt, pepper (to taste)

Directions:

Create a paste with beans and oats by pulsing in food processor. In a large mixing bowl, combine paste with remaining ingredient list. Using wet hands, form the mixture into a burger shape. Add one tablespoon of olive oil to frying pan and heat over medium. Cook burgers on each side 7 minutes, until brown and crispy.

Fennel and Beetroot Burger

Preparation time: 10 minutes Cooking time: 50 minutes
Servings 6–8 burgers

Ingredients:

2 medium size beetroots, peeled and grated

2 tablespoons chopped dill

1 fennel bulb, trimmed and finely chopped

1 cup cooked brown rice

2 tablespoons cornmeal

1/4 cup tomato sauce

Salt, pepper (tp taste)

Directions:

In a large mixing bowl, combine grated beets, fennel, dill, brown rice and cornmeal. Stir in the tomato sauce, salt/pepper, form small patties. Add one tablespoon of olive oil to frying pan and fry burger for 6 minutes on each side. Serve on vegan burger buns and favorite toppings

Sautéed Green Beans, Mushrooms & Tomatoes

Preparation Time: 15 minutes Cooking Time: 15 minutes

Servings: 10

Ingredients:

Water 3 lb. green beans, trimmed

2 tablespoons olive oil

8 cloves garlic, minced

½ cup tomato, diced

12 oz. cremini mushrooms, sliced into quarters

Salt and pepper to taste

Directions:

Fill a pot with water. Bring to a boil. Add the beans and cook for 5 minutes. Drain the beans. Dry the pot. Pour oil into the pot. Add garlic, tomato and mushrooms. Cook for 5 minutes. Add the beans and cook for another 5 minutes. Season with salt and pepper. Store in a food container and reheat before eating.

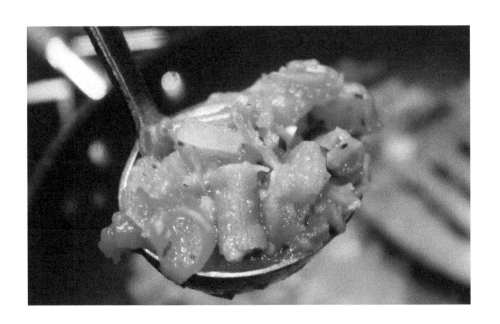

Green Beans, Roasted Red Peppers & Onions

Preparation Time: 15 minutes Cooking Time: 25 minutes
Servings: 6

Ingredients:

1 tablespoon olive oil

1 ½ cups onion, chopped

1 tablespoon red wine vinegar

½ cup jarred roasted red peppers, drained and chopped

2 tablespoons fresh basil, chopped

¼ cup olives, pitted and sliced Salt and pepper to taste

1 lb. fresh green beans, trimmed and sliced

Directions:

Pour olive oil in a pan over medium heat. Add onion and cook for 10 minutes. Pour in the vinegar. Cook for 2 minutes. Add roasted red peppers, basil and olives. Season with salt and pepper. Remove from the stove. In a saucepan with water, cook beans for 10 minutes. Add beans to the onion mixture. Stir for 3 minutes.

Sweet Spicy Beans

Preparation Time: 10 minutes Cooking Time: 50 minutes

Servings: 10

Ingredients:

3 tablespoons vegetable oil

1 onion, chopped

45 oz. navy beans, rinsed and drained

1 ½ cups water

¾ cup ketchup

⅓ cup brown sugar

1 tablespoon white vinegar

1 teaspoon chipotle peppers in adobo sauce

Salt and pepper to taste

Directions:

Pour the oil in a pan over medium heat. Add onion and cook for 10 minutes. Add the rest of the Ingredients. Bring to a boil. Reduce heat and simmer for 30 minutes. Transfer to food container. Reheat when ready to eat.

Creamy Veggie Risotto

Preparation time: 15 minutes Cooking time: 35 minutes
Servings: 4

Ingredients:

2 Tablespoons Olive Oil

1 Clove Garlic, Minced

½ Sweet Onion, Diced

1 Bunch Asparagus Tips, Chopped into 1 Inch Pieces

2 ¾ Cups Vegetable Stock

1 Cup Arborio Rice, Rinsed & Drained

1 Teaspoon Thyme, Dried

1 Cup Sugar Snap Peas, Trimmed & Rinsed

Sea Sal t& Black Pepper to Taste

Pinch Red Pepper Flakes

2 Tablespoons Vegan Butter

2 Cups Baby Spinach, Fresh & Torn

½ Lemon, Juiced

Directions:

Press sauté and set it to low, and then add in your oil. Once it's hot cook your onion for two minutes, stirring often. Add in the asparagus and garlic, cooking for another thirty seconds. Add in the salt, pepper, red pepper flakes, thyme, stock and rice. Stir well and then seal the lid. Cook on high pressure for eight minutes. Use a quick release, and then stir in your vegan butter, spinach, and lemon juice. Stir and serve warm.

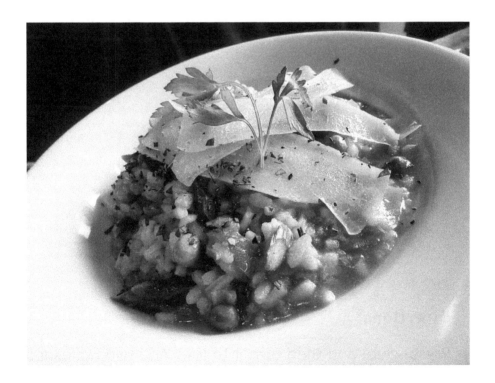

Leek & Mushroom Risotto

Preparation time: 10 minutes Cooking time: 50 minutes

Servings: 4

Ingredients:

4 Tablespoons Vegan Butter, Divided

1 Leek, Sliced

12 Ounces Baby Bella Mushrooms, Sliced

1 Cup Arborio Rice, Rinsed & Drained

2 Cloves Garlic, Minced

2 ¾ Cup Vegetable Stock

1 Teaspoon Thyme

½ Lemon, Juiced Sea

Salt & Black Pepper to Taste

Parsley, Fresh & Chopped for Garnish

Directions:

Press sauté and then turn it to low. Add two tablespoons of butter, and once it's melted add in your mushrooms and leek. Sauté for two minutes, and stir often. Add in your garlic, cooking for thirty seconds. Throw in the rice, cooking for one minute and stirring often to toast it. turn it off of sauté. Stir in your salt, thyme and stock. Close the lid, and cook on high pressure for eight minutes. Use a quick release. Add lemon juice and two tablespoons of vegan butter, and then season with salt and pepper. Garnish with parsley before serving.

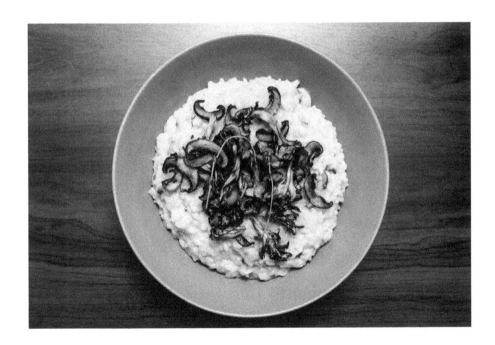

Cabbage Roll Bowls

Preparation time: 10 minutes Cooking time: 40 minutes Servings: 6

Ingredients:

Tempeh: 1 Tablespoon Olive Oil

8 Ounces Tempeh, Crumbled

2 Teaspoon Montreal Steak Seasoning

2 Cloves Garlic, Minced

2 Teaspoons Vegan Worcestershire Sauce

1 Bay Leaf

½ Onion, Diced Cabbage

Rolls: 1 Cup Basmati Rice, Rinsed & Drained

1 Cup Water

1 ½ Cups Vegetable Stock Sea

Salt & Black Pepper to Tate

1 Head Cabbage, Sliced Thin

6 Ounces Tomato Paste

½ Teaspoon Paprika Pinch Cayenne

Pepper ¼ Cup Parsley, Fresh & Chopped

Directions:

Select sauté and make sure it's set to low. Once your instant pot is hot, add in your oil. When your oil begins to shimmer, add in the tempeh with Montreal steak seasoning, garlic, bay leaf, Worcestershire shire sauce and onion. Cook for four minutes, and then place it in a bowl. Set the bowl to the side. Clean your instant pot and then add in your water, salt and rice. Lock the lid, and then cook on high pressure for eight minutes with the lid sealed. Allow for a natural pressure release for ten minutes before following with a quick release. Fluff the rice, and add in the cabbage, tomato paste, stock, paprika, pepper and cayenne. Press sauté and select low. Cook for five minutes. Your cabbage should soften, and then discard the bay leaf. Stir in your parsley, and serve warm with tempeh.

Coconut Rice & Veggies

Preparation time: 10 minutes Cooking time: 30 minutes

Servings: 4

Ingredients:

1 Cup Jasmine Rice, Rinsed & Drained

1 Cup Water

1 Cup Bok Choy, Chopped

1 Carrot, Sliced

1 Onion, Small & Deiced

1 Tablespoon Sesame Oil

½ Teaspoon Ground Ginger

Sea Salt & Black Pepper to Taste

1 Cup Sugar Snap Peas, Rinsed & Trimmed

8 Ounces Water Chestnuts, Canned, Sliced & Drained

2 Cloves Garlic, Minced

8 Ounces White Button Mushrooms, Sliced

14 Ounces Coconut Milk, Canned & Lite

1 Teaspoon Chinese Five Spice

1 Teaspoon Soy Sauce

Directions: Combine your water, salt, ginger and rice. Lock the lid and cook on high pressure for four minutes. Use a natural pressure release for five minutes before following with a quick release. Fluff the rice, and then place it in a bowl. Set the rice to the side. Press sauté and select low, and then add in your oil. Once it's hot add in the carrot, bok choy, snap peas, onion, garlic, mushrooms and water chestnuts. Cook for three minutes. Stir in the five-spice powder, soy sauce, coconut milk and cooked rice. Allow it to simmer for six minutes and serve warm. The coconut milk should reduce.

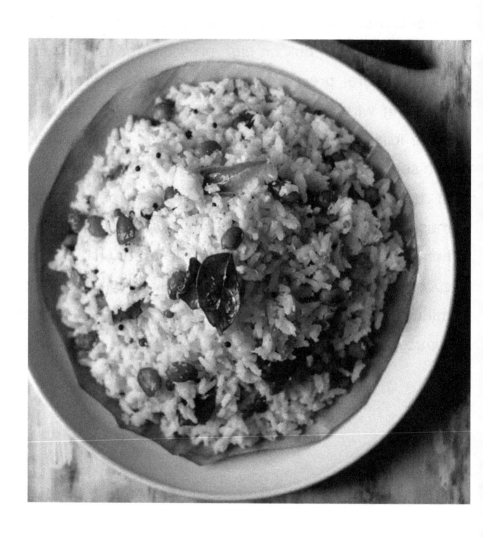

Quinoa & Butternut Chili

Preparation time: 10 minutes Cooking time: 40 minutes

Servings: 4

Ingredients:

2 Tablespoons Olive Oil

2 Carrots, Sliced

1 Red Bell Pepper, Diced

1 Sweet Onion, Diced

1 Jalapeno Pepper, Diced

2 Cloves Garlic, Minced

1 Butternut Squash, Peeled & Cubed

14 Ounces Diced Tomatoes, Canned & With Juices

1 Cup Quinoa, Rinsed

1 Bay Leaf

1 Teaspoon Cumin

2 ½ Cups Vegetable Stock

Sea Salt & Black Pepper to Taste

½ Teaspoon Chili Powder

½ Teaspoon Sweet Paprika

1 Teaspoon Cumin

1 Tablespoon Lemon Juice, Fresh

Directions: Press sauté, and then add in your oil. Once your oil is hot add in the jalapeno, bell pepper, carrots and onion. Cook for three minutes, and stir often. Turn it off of sauté, and then add in your garlic. Stir and cook for thirty seconds. Add your tomatoes, quinoa, stock bay leaf, squash, cumin, salt, paprika, chili powder and pepper. Seal the lid, and cook on high pressure for eight minutes. Use a natural pressure release for ten minutes, and then use a quick release. Discard the bay leaf before stirring in your lemon juice. Season with salt and pepper if desired. If it is too liquid, press sauté and cook for two minutes more.

Vegan Pad Thai

Preparation time: 10 minutes Cooking time: 40 minutes
Servings: 2

Ingredients:

Sauce:

½ Tablespoons Ginger, Fresh & Minced

2 Cloves Garlic, Minced

1 Teaspoon Sesame Oil

1 Teaspoon Maple Syrup

 2 Teaspoons Sriracha

1 ½ Cups Water

½ Cup Vegetable Broth

2 Teaspoons

Sushi Grain Meal

Preparation Time: 20 minutes Cooking Time: 0 minute

Servings: 4

Ingredients:

2 teaspoons fresh ginger, grated

2 tablespoons low sodium tamari

2 tablespoons rice vinegar

2 teaspoons sesame oil, toasted

2 tablespoons avocado oil

2 cups brown rice, cooked

1 cup cucumber, diced

1 cup carrot, shredded

1 avocado, diced

1 cup toasted nori, chopped

1 cup shelled edamame, cooked

Sesame seeds

Directions:

In a bowl, mix the ginger, tamari, vinegar, sesame oil and avocado oil. Divide brown rice among 4 food containers with lids. Top with the cucumber, carrot, avocado, nori and edamame. Sprinkle sesame seeds on top. Seal the container and refrigerate. Drizzle sauce on top when ready to eat.

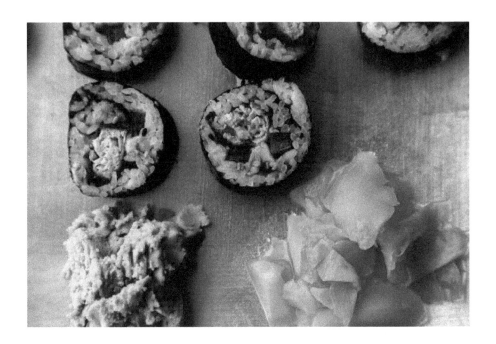

Quinoa & Snap Pea Salad

Preparation Time: 20 minutes Cooking Time: 20 minutes Servings: 6

Ingredients:

2 cups water

1 cup quinoa

⅓ cup onion, sliced

1 ½ cups mushrooms, sliced

1 tablespoon fresh dill, chopped

2 cups fresh snap peas, trimmed and sliced

⅓ cup white wine vinegar

¼ cup flaxseed oil

1 teaspoon lemon zest

1 tablespoon lemon juice

1 teaspoon maple syrup

Directions:

Put quinoa and water in a pan over medium high heat. Bring to a boil. Reduce heat and simmer for 15 minutes. Fluff using a fork and set aside. In a bowl, combine onion, mushrooms, dill and peas. In another bowl, mix the rest of the Ingredients. Transfer the quinoa in a food container. Stir in the pea mixture. Seal the container and refrigerate until ready to serve. Transfer the maple dressing into a glass jar with lid. Drizzle dressing over the quinoa salad before serving.

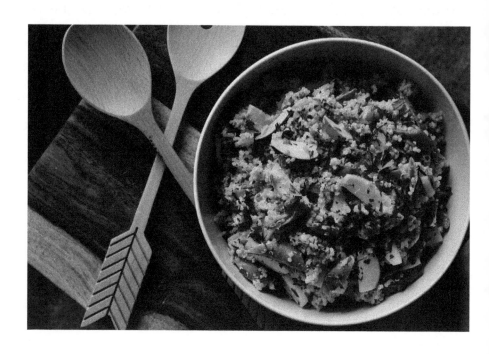

Chickpea & Quinoa

Preparation Time: 15 minutes Cooking Time: 0 minute
Serving: 1

Ingredients:

3 tablespoons hummus

1 tablespoon lemon juice

1 tablespoon roasted red pepper, chopped

1 tablespoon water Salt and pepper to taste

1 cup cooked quinoa

¼ avocado, diced

⅓ cup canned chickpeas, rinsed and drained

½ cup cherry tomatoes, sliced in half

½ cup cucumber, sliced

Directions:

In a glass jar with lid, mix the hummus, lemon juice, red
pepper, water, salt and pepper. Shake to mix. Arrange

the rest of the Ingredients in a food container. Drizzle
with sauce when ready to eat.

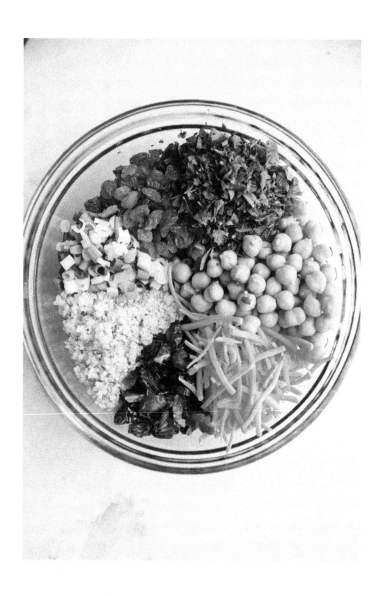

Black Beans with Rice

Preparation Time: 20 minutes Cooking Time: 2 hours and 15 minutes Servings: 8

Ingredients:

1 lb. dried black beans, soaked in water overnight, rinsed and drained

8 cups water, divided

2 tablespoons dried oregano

1 bay leaf

6 cloves garlic, crushed

2 teaspoons olive oil

1 onion, chopped

1 red bell pepper, chopped

1 tablespoon ground cumin

1 jalapeño pepper, chopped

2 tablespoons balsamic vinegar

Salt and pepper to taste

2 cups long-grain white rice

8 lime wedges

Directions: Put black beans in a pot. Add 4 cups water, oregano, bay leaf and garlic. Bring to a boil. Reduce heat and simmer for 2 hours. Drain and put beans back to the pot. Pour in the oil. Add onion and bell pepper. Cook for 5 minutes. Add jalapeño pepper and cumin. Cook for 1 minute. Season with salt and pepper. In another saucepan, add remaining water and salt. Add rice and cover. Bring to a boil and then simmer for 15 minutes. Put rice in a food container and top with beans. Garnish with lemon wedges. Refrigerate and then reheat before serving.

Slow Cooked Beans

Preparation Time: 10 minutes Cooking Time: 2 hours and 15 minutes Servings: 4

Ingredients:

1 lb. black beans, soaked overnight, rinsed and drained

1 onion, chopped

1 bay leaf

4 cloves garlic, minced

1 teaspoon dried thyme

 5 cups boiling water

Salt to taste

Directions:

Add the beans to a slow cooker. Stir in onion, bay leaf, garlic and thyme. Add water and cover the pot. Cook for 2 hours. Season with salt and cook for another 15 minutes.

Mango with Quinoa & Black Beans

Preparation Time: 30 minutes Cooking Time: 30 minutes
Servings: 2

Ingredients:

½ cup quinoa, toasted

1 cup water

¼ cup orange juice

¼ cup fresh cilantro, chopped

2 tablespoons rice vinegar

2 teaspoons sesame oil, toasted

1 teaspoon fresh ginger, minced

Salt to taste Cayenne pepper to taste

1 mango, diced

1 red bell pepper, diced

1 cup canned black beans

2 scallions, sliced thinly

Directions:

Put quinoa in a pot. Pour in water. Bring to a boil. Reduce heat to simmer for 20 minutes. While waiting, mix the rest of the Ingredients. Add the quinoa to the mango mixture and transfer to a food container. Refrigerate for up to 2 days. Serve chilled.

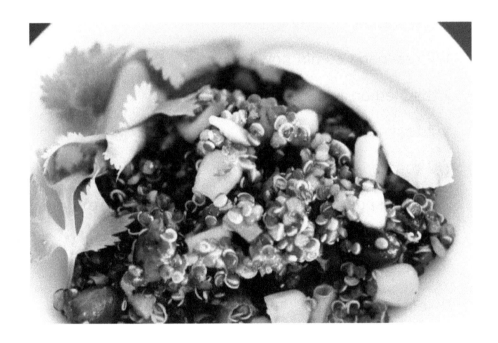

Roasted Red Pepper Hummus

Preparation Time: 30minutes

Ingredients:

15.5 oz canned chickpeas (washed and drained)

1 clove of garlic

2 tbsp tahini

1/2 teaspoon cumin powder

2 tbsp lemon juice

1/2 teaspoon of sea salt

1/2 roasted red pepper

2-3 tablespoons of water (if necessary to dilute) (you can also use extra virgin olive oil if desired)

Directions:

With the food processor running, put the garlic clove and process until minced. If you want to tune a little, drizzle a few tablespoons of water (or oil if desired) on top of the food processor while it is running. Use as a pasta for sandwiches or as a sauce for vegetables, crackers or chips. Yum!

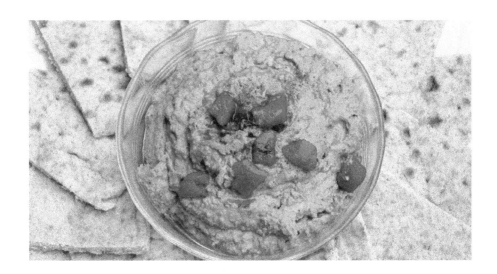

Queso

Preparation Time: 30minutes

Ingredients:

1 1/2 cups pumpkin (peeled and sown before dicing - or you can buy a pack of pre-sliced pumpkin)

1/2 cup raw cashew nuts

1 tbsp fresh lemon juice

1/2 teaspoon smoked paprika

2 tbsp Nutritional yeast

1/2 teaspoon salt

1/2 teaspoon saffron

1 tin of 4.5 oz diced green peppers

Directions:

Add the diced squash and cashews in a pan and cover with water for at least 1 inch. Bring to a boil, lower the heat to med and cook for about 20 minutes until the pumpkin is tender. When the pumpkin/cashews are ready, drain and pour into a high-speed blender. Add lemon juice, smoked paprika, Nutritional yeast, salt and turmeric. Mix until completely smooth by adding nondairy milk (or water) 1 tbsp at a time to move things around if necessary. You will need to use the tamper to push the INGREDIENTS to the bottom. Do not do too thin! Use just enough liquid to mix everything. I used about 3-4 tablespoons. When completely smooth, pour the mixture into a pan (you can use the same one you used for pumpkin/cashews) and mix in the parsley and chopped green peppers. Gently heat the queso over medium heat until thickened and bubbling. Serve immediately with Tortilla Chips.

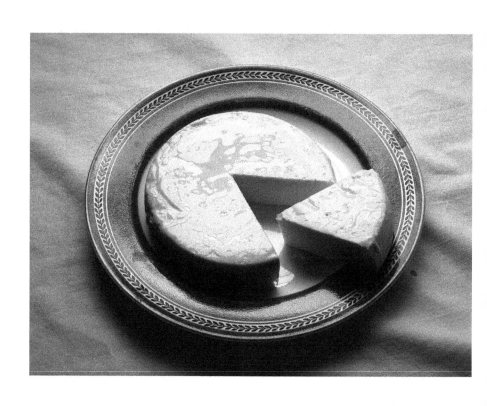

Sweet Potato and Bean Burgers

Preparation time: 10 minutes Cooking time: 30 minutes

Servings 8–10 burgers

Ingredients:

3 cups cannellini white beans, drained

2 sweet potatoes, peeled, boiled and mashed

3 tablespoons tahini paste

1 teaspoon Cajun seasoning

1/3 cup whole wheat flour

Salt, pepper to taste

Directions:

Puree the beans in a food processor until smooth. In a large mixing bowl combine beans with mashed potatoes and stir. Add the rest of the ingredient list and mix well. Using wet hands, form the mixture into a burger shape. Add one tablespoon of olive oil to frying pan and heat over medium. Cook burgers on each side 4 minutes, until golden brown. Serve with your choice of bread, toppings, and condiments.

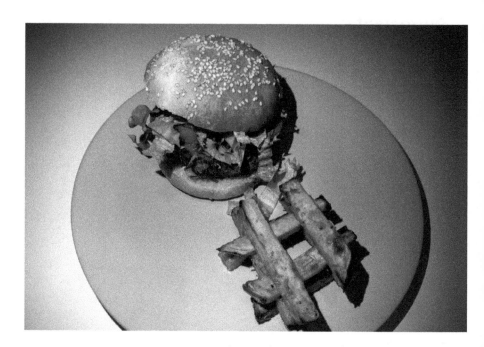

Lightning Source UK Ltd.
Milton Keynes UK
UKHW021830161222
414027UK00001B/17